Anti-Inflammatory Diet Guide to Fight Inflammation with 36 Easy Recipes

By Rebecca Publishing

Anti-Inflammatory Diet Guide to Fight Inflammation with 36 Easy Recipes by Rebecca Publishing

Disclaimer

Anti-Inflammatory Diet Guide to Fight Inflammation with 36 Easy Recipes by Rebecca Publishing

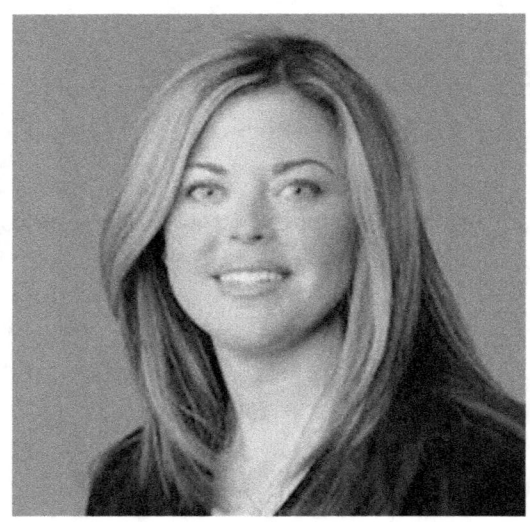

About the author!

I am a newbie to publishing business, but I have a lot of information to tell you. I have been studying healthy way of eating from leading nutritionist in Europe and I have a lot of useful information on this topic. I have lost more than 20 kilos so I can provide you with a lot of practical tips on this matter.

My story is also very bright, after giving birth to a child; I have gained a lot of extra weight. It was simply impossible to look into the mirror, but I decided to do my best to return to my previous shape. I have tried swimming, jogging, different diets like Dukan, Sugar Free Diet, Kremlyovskaya Diet etc. These diets forced me to starving and nothing more. I saw and fell the best result after following the Paleo Diet. This diet helped me to loose ALL my extra weight this is more than 20 kilos/44 pounds and I feel myself much healthier now! So, I am glad to share with you 57 of my beloved paleo recipes, I hope you will find them healthy and delicious as well.

Introduction

Thank you for downloading of my Anti-Inflammatory Diet Guide to Fight Inflammation with 36 Easy Recipes. I studied carefully this information over the best books on Inflammation, also I was consulting several nutritionists before writing this guide. I hope you will enjoy it and it will help you.

Table of Content

Anti-inflammatory diet: the way to be healthy?

"You are what you eat" – this phrase rings truer than you think. Just look in your refrigerator and you will see enormous number of junk foods and drinks which cause inflammation and diseases in your body. Below you will see some examples of bad habits and unhealthy foods you eat every day.

- high amounts of sugar and corn syrups which is rich in fructose can lead to insulin resistance syndrome, diabetes and overweight;

- an excessive amount of refined carbohydrates (white bread) can cause inflammation, insulin resistance syndrome and obesity;

- processed and vacuum-packaged foods that contain additives and trans fats are causing inflammation and damage the endothelial cells;

- vegetable oils are harmful to health. Regular vegetable oils ingestion becomes the reason of Omega-6 to Omega-3 fatty acids misbalance which in turn leads to inflammatory processes in the body;

- Excessive drinking can make you lose control of your own life. It is a very bad habit. Just break yourself of it!

- excessive intake of processed meat leads to strong inflammatory effects in the body;

- little physical activity can also drive inflammation.

To avoid all these health problems - choose Anti-inflammatory Diet!

This diet gives you more long lasting results than anti-inflammatory medication. Taking anti-inflammatory medications, you start to feel much better in a short space of time. As for the anti-inflammatory diet, it will require more of your patience. But in a few weeks you will espy a significant difference in symptoms. It is proved that Anti-inflammatory Diet is unprovable for strengthening overall health. It can reduce cardiovascular diseases, regulate blood triglyceride and tension of blood, calm patients with arthritis joints.

Anti-inflammatory Diet – is a healthy diet that reduces not only the risk of long-term illness but improves your mood and living standards! It is enriched with fruits, vegetables, nuts, whole grains, fish, healthy oils!

This diet was developed by the Harvard-educated professor and pioneer in integrative medicine - Andrew Weil. According to Dr. Weil's researches, certain foods are able to inhibit inflammatory processes in the human organism. He proposes to serve up only healthy fats, lots of water, fiber-rich vegetables and fruits, oily fish and limited number of animal protein.

The Anti-Inflammatory Diet includes daily consumption of 2000 to 3000 calories, according to size, gender and level of activity. 40-50% of calories you get from carbohydrates, 30% - from fat and 20-30% - from protein. Dr.Weil recommends to mix all three nutrients at each meal.

As Dr Weil says, Anti-inflammatory Diet is based on the Mediterranean Diet but have several extras: dark chocolate and green tea. It provides for the use of a great number of fresh foods, especially fruits and vegetables because they provide phytonutrients that combat cancer cells and other degenerative diseases. A huge role is played by consumption of Omega 3 fatty acids and limiting fast foods, fried products at all costs.

So this way of eating helps to avoid chronic inflammatory processes and it will fill your body with essential fatty acids, energy, minerals, fiber, vitamins and make you slimmer.

What is inflammation and how to reduce inflammatory processes in you body using the Anti-inflammatory Diet?

Anti-Inflammatory Diet Guide to Fight Inflammation with 36 Easy Recipes by Rebecca Publishing

Experts define inflammation as a localized reaction of tissues to irritation, injury or infection. The symptoms of inflammation are tiredness, pain, redness of area, swelling, sweating, burning and heat and sometimes loss of movement.

Inflammation causes variety of different serious maladies. But you can challenge inflammatory processes. Just choose an Anti-Inflammation Diet to control inflammation in your body.

But there is one more type of inflammation - chronic inflammation. It is a natural process which makes your immune system to work at full capacity to remove the source of its origin as soon as possible.

Besides, sometimes because of stress, poor nutrition, genetic predisposition, toxins, the lack or absence of exercises our body can have chronic inflammation without apparent reasons. As a result, the person becomes vulnerable to dangerous diseases such as cancer, neurodegenerative diseases, cardiovascular diseases etc. However, Anti-inflammatory foods and the diet can solve this problem and weaken symptoms.

Health Benefits of the Anti-Inflammation Diet

Proven for use that diet has a beneficial effect on human health:

- Heart disease: body uses fatty deposits for damaged arteries recovery.
- Cancer: fresh healthy fruits and green vegetables, proteins significantly decrease the chances of getting cancer
- Arthritis and joint pain: Arthritis is the constant companion of inflammation. But thanks to Anti-Inflammation Diet it is possible to ease the pain and postpone the onset. The secret is in fresh, natural, healthy vitamin-rich foods.

- Weight gain: one more companion of inflammation – is obesity. It increases inflammation in the organism but right foods can reduce inflammation and thereby influence on your kilos. Reducing inflammation induces weight loss!

Basic principles of an Anti-inflammatory Diet

So, if you are seeking a healthy diet start with an Anti-inflammatory Diet! Your condition depends on your diet! Just choose a diet of anti-inflammatory foods and you will understand that you can resist inflammatory diseases.

Here are some principals of an Anti-inflammatory Diet you need to know:

- eat anti-inflammatory foods enriched with Omega 3 fatty acids
- remove processed foods
- choose only organic fruits and vegetables that are enriched with inflammation-reducing antioxidants
- take right herbs and spices to combat inflammation
- exclude unhealthy fats and foods causing allergies
- get enough sleep

Follow these simple basic principals and turn your mind to what you can eat instead of what you can't.

Foods to Avoid

Here is the list of some pro-inflammatory foods. You`d better to avoid these products or eliminate from your diet-menu.

- Beverages: latte, coffee, fizzy soda drinks, fruit juice, black tea
- Refined carbohydrates: white pasta, white bread, white rice, white potatoes, refined sugar, flour and foods enriched with glycemic index
- Desserts: sugary cereals and candies, cookies, cakes, pastries
- Processed meat: bologna, red meat, hot dogs, sausages, etc.
- Diary: frozen yogurt, butter, peanut butter, cheese, ice-cream
- Processed foods: crackers, chips and pretzels (because these foods contain additives and food coloring).
- Certain oils: corn, sunflower, safflower, peanut oil, soybean oil.
- Alcohol: alcohol in large quantities
- Some vegetables: potatoes, tomatoes, eggplants, peppers because they contain a chemical alkaloid named solanine - that can cause pain
- Trans fats: processed foods, fast foods, margarine, coffee creamers, donuts, crackers, cookies, cheeseburgers, pizza

Foods to Eat

Here is the list of foods that can prevent inflammation:

- Vegetables: Brussels sprouts, broccoli, cabbage, cauliflower, spinach, celery, beets
- Fruit: grapes, cherries. blackberries, raspberries are inflammation fighters; pineapple
- Beverages: green tea, chamomile tea, clean water; cabbage, spinach, cucumbers, fennel, lemon, ginger juices, coconut milk, red vine
- High-fat fruits: olives and avocados

- Healthy fats: coconut oil, olive oil, avocado oil

- Fatty fish: herring, mackerel and anchovies, tuna, sardines, salmon

- Nuts & seeds: celery seeds, almonds, walnuts, chia seeds, flaxseeds

- Peppers: bell pepper and chili pepper, cayenne pepper

- Chocolate: black chocolate

- Herbs &Spices: garlic, turmeric, ginger and cinnamon, chili, ginger, oregano, rosemary, black pepper and anise (contain bioflavonoids and polyphenols, limit free radical production)

- Soy products: tempeh, tofu, soy milk, beans

- Whole grains: oatmeal, brown rice

- Carbohydrates: rye bread, brown rice, wholegrain pasta

- Eggs: organic pasteurized eggs

All you need to know about "BAD" and "GOOD" fats when you are on an Anti-inflammatory Diet

When you are on an an Anti-inflammatory Diet it does not mean that you should avoid eating fats. It is not forbidden! But you should know which fats are "GOOD" and which are "BAD". Despite the fact that fats cause revulsion in many people and are associated with excess weight, they play an important role in a healthy lifestyle:

Good fats: polyunsaturated and monounsaturated fats, the omega-3 fatty acids
Not friendly fats: saturated fats
Bad fats: trans fats

Now you know almost everything about an anti-inflammatory Diet: you know what foods you should choose to prevent or reduce inflammation. But what methods of cooking are preferable for this diet? We need only healthy anti-inflammatory methods to keep all the benefits of products

- Baking: use the oven to bake foods. You may bake vegetables, fish, meat in its natural juices using ceramic and glass baking dish.
- Steaming: use a steamer to cook any food you like. Marinate meat, fish, vegetables, sea food with spices and herbs and than steam but do not overcook. As a result, you will enjoy a flavorful healthy dish.
- Poaching: for this gentle method of cooking you will need poaching liquid. Just boil water and put any food you like in the boiled water. Cook until tender and flavored broth use as a base for soup.
- Stir-frying: if you choose this method of cooking, you will need a small amount of oil. Fry meat or vegetables at high temperatures for a very short time.
- Grilling and broiling: this method is the best for fish and vegetables but not for meat. Because of high temperatures proteins in meat turn into *heterocyclic amines*, which are very harmful for your body and may cause different types of cancer.
- Microwaving: despite the fact that this method is very fast it is unsuitable for cooking healthy food. Due to the high temperature destroys all the nutrients. That is why you should avoid this cooking method in your practice.

An Anti-Inflammatory Diet Sample Menu Plan

Breakfast

- omelet with mushrooms and kale, fried in coconut oil.

- cherries (or any berries you like).

- a cup of green tea or still water (or homemade smoothie).

Lunch

- grilled fish with greens, olive oil and vinegar.

- raspberries covered   with plain Greek yogurt (or non-dairy yogurt) and chopped nuts

- tea with ice cubes or water.

Snack

- bell pepper with guacamole.

Dinner

- chicken curry with cauliflower or broccoli.

- red wine (140–280 g).

- dark chocolate or a cup of melted dark chocolate

Some facts about the beneficial properties of herbs and spices

An Anti-inflammatory Diet is intimately connected with intake of herbs and spices. We can't imagine any dish, beverage or sauce without these "fragrant friends". Their healthy and nutritional properties are so great and powerful that nutritionists can`t think how they struggled with inflammatory processes in the body.

Turmeric (Curcumin)

Curcumin is a yellow pigment which is contained in turmeric. It has an anti-inflammatory effect, prevent inflammation and treat wounds, infections and resolves digestive problems. It is a powerful antioxidant that even fight cancer.

Green tea

Confess, every one of you drink green tea and is familiar with its smooth taste and energizing effect! But in addition, green tea has a positive anti-inflammatory effect. It prevents cardio-vascular conditions and cancer; it also treats arthritis. If you have problems with digestion, drink 3-4 cups of fragrant green tea a day! This wonderful drink reduce inflammation and will soothe the pain.

Chili Peppers (Capsaicin)

There are variety of red hot chili peppers but all they are united by chemical capsaicin. It makes pepper hot and creates an anti-inflammatory effect, fights cancer, aids weight loss and strengthens immunity.

Include in your menu different types of chili peppers cayenne or jalapeno, they also contain capsaicin. Enjoy healthy chili dishes!

Black Pepper

Black pepper contains chemical piperine. Any dose of this substance, even the smallest can reduce pain, inflammation and arthritis symptoms.

Rosemary

Rosemary fights with inflammation and oxidation. Chop it and add in your salads, soups and other dishes. Try healthy and useful properties of this herb!

Ginger

Doctors and nutritionists say that ginger has a powerful therapeutic influence and treats pain and inflammation better than non-steroidal anti-inflammatory drugs.

This spice helps relieve the symptoms of nausea, prevents vomiting due to sickness, pregnancy and after chemotherapy. It is recommended for heart diseases, nausea, flu and cold.

Cinnamon

Cinnamon is extracted from the bark of cinnamon trees. This spice has antibacterial, antioxidant, ant carcinogenic and lipid-lowering properties. It relieves neurological disorders such as Alzheimer's and Parkinson's diseases, improves brain function, supports weight loss, combats diabetes, treats digestion.

Nutmeg

Nutmeg contains myristicin that helps to reduce cholesterol. The extract of nutmeg kills leukemia cells and has rejuvenating action on human skin. Compounds contained in nutmeg protects skin from the sun's UV rays. Include nutmeg in your diet and it improves your memory, calms the symptoms of anxiety, kills rotavirus infection.

And that's not the whole list of useful properties of nutmeg.

Garlic

Known to all, ordinary garlic, which is so not like the children and many adults because of its pungent smell. But do you know that garlic

- prevents cardio-vascular conditions
- reduces inflammation
- protects arteries against inflammation
- reduces blood fats and cholesterol
- improves blood circulation and cardiac work
- stimulates immunological system of human body
- fights against infections, flu and cold
- has great effect against worms
- improves digestion
- relieves the symptoms of skin diseases such as psoriasis

Cilantro

This green herb is rich in magnesium, fiber, iron, rich. It is a perfect antioxidant.

Cilantro in any of its form helps the digestive system, cleans the body and removes heavy metals, toxins from the body, regulates blood sugar, stimulates immunological system and endocrine glands, eases rheumatoid disease.

Basil and Mint

First of all, basil is one of the powerful herbal allies. It contains eugenol, compound that reduces inflammation in the body. Basil It has many "anti" effects: anti-inflammatory, ant carcinogenic, antiseptic, anti-fungal and other anti- effects. Basil supports digestive system, relieves nausea, colitis.

Mint is a fragrant herb, excellent antiseptic with calming, relaxing and anti-inflammatory effects.

Cloves

Cloves also contain eugenol which blocks the cyclooxygenase - the main causative agent of inflammatory processes in the body

This spice controls cardiac work, cancerous diseases and has antifungal effect.

Oregano

Oregano contains beta-caryophyllin, the substance that slows inflammation. It is mostly used by people suffering from osteoporosis and rheumatic arteriosclerosis.

It also has bactericidal and antifungal impact. Additionally, oregano has antioxidant effect that stimulates immunological system and prevents cancer.

Sage

Sage is the herb that has a lot of health benefits. It is known as natural anti-inflammatory. It relieves menstrual molimina, improves circulation of the blood, kills microbes and bacteria.

Drink sage tea, add sage leaves to your dishes, create your own recipes and the payoff comes in due time!

Thyme

Thyme is rich in nutrients and widely used for medicinal purposes.

Here is the list of sage health benefits:

- improves digestion and mood
- prevents inflammation
- stimulates immunological system of human body
- fights against infections

RECIPES OF DISHES FOR AN ANTI-INFLAMMATORY DIET BREAKFAST (LUNCH)

1. Cherry coconut porridge

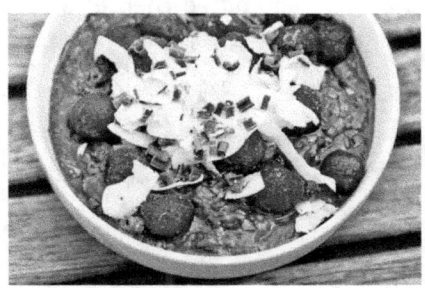

INGREDIENTS

Oats – 300 gr

Fresh or frozen pitted cherries

Chia seed – four tbsp.

Coconut milk – 1 l

Raw cacao – 75 gr

Stevia – 0,5 tsp.

Coconut chips

Black chocolate shavings

Maple syrup

INSTRUCTIONS

1. Take 300 gr of oats, 1 l of coconut milk, 75 gr of raw cacao, four tbsp. of chia seeds and 0,5 tsp. of stevia and mix all ingredients in a saucepan.

2. Boil your porridge on slow fire up to readiness.

3. Pour the ready porridge into a bowl, add pitted cherries and sprinkle with coconut chips, grated chocolate and maple syrup.

4. Enjoy your cherry coconut porridge

2. Overnight oatmeal

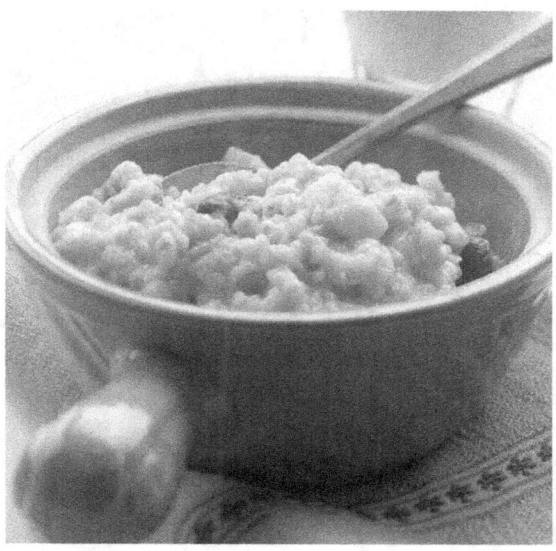

INGREDIENTS

Oats – 47 gr

Puree of 1 banana

Almond milk – 240 ml

Chia seeds – 50 gr

Vanilla extract – 2 gr

INSTRUCTIONS

1.Combine oats, banana puree, almond milk, chia seeds and vanilla extract together in a big container and put into the refrigerator for 12 hours or overnight.

2. Serve cold.

3. Zucchini Pizza

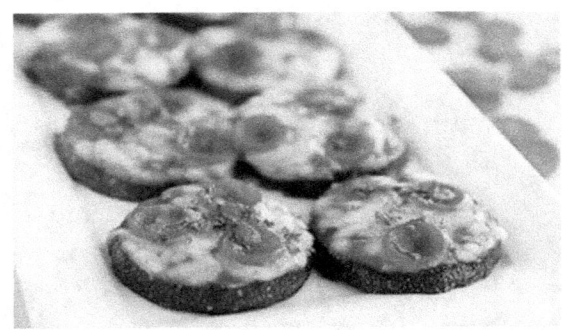

INGREDIENTS

Zucchini – 1 piece

Mozzarella

Parmesan

Olive oil

Pizza Sauce

<u>Herbs and spices</u>

Salt

Pepper

Dried Oregano

Fresh basil

INSTRUCTIONS

1. Shred Mozzarella and parmesan. Chop fresh basil.

2. Slice zucchini in circles. Sprinkle each circle with olive oil, salt and pepper.

3. Fry on both sides until golden brown. Put shredded mozzarella, pizza sauce, dried oregano and basil on top of fried zucchini.

4. Cover and cook for two more minutes..

5. Drizzle with shredded parmesan.

6. Serve and enjoy!

4. Roasted Beets and Feta

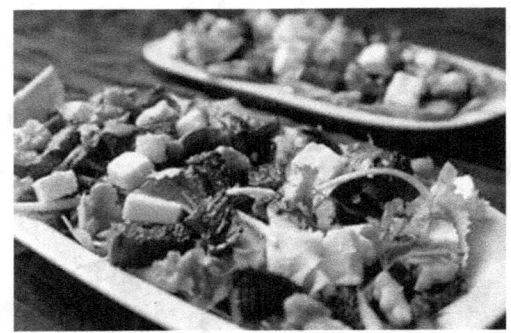

INGREDIENTS

Beets – 4-5pcs

Olive oil

Sweet onion – 1 piece

Clove of garlic – 2 pcs

Feta

INSTRUCTIONS

1.Peel and quarter beets. Put beet chunks into a bowl.

2.Turn on the oven and preheat to 175 C. Grease the baking sheet with oil.

3.Toss beet chunks with olive oil and move to a baking dish.

4.Bake for an hour.

5. Meanwhile, mix chopped onion with feta cheese.

5. Cool beets and serve with feta-onion sauce.

5. Spirulina and Cilantro Guacamole

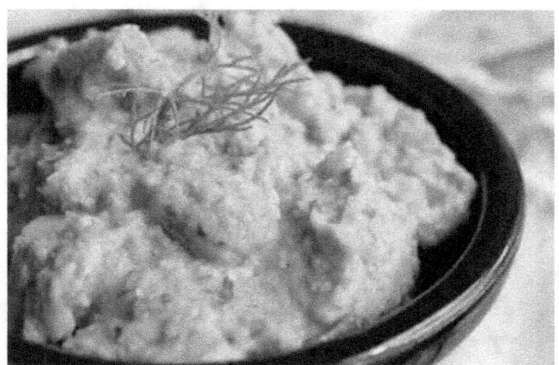

INGREDIENTS

Avocado – 1 piece

Juice of one lemon

Garlic bulbets – 2 pcs

Onion – 1 piece

Tomato – 1 piece

Fresh cilantro -1 cup

Spirulina – 25 gr

Salt and pepper

INSTRUCTIONS

1. Before cooking prepare ingredients: wash and dry vegetables, hop garlic, onion and fresh cilantro. Cut tomato into small cubes.

2. Make avocado puree and add lemon juice. Mix.

3. Add chopped vegetables to the avocado mixture.

4. Blend carefully and add25 gr of spirulina

5. Season with salt and pepper.

6. Creamy Lemon, Garlic and Onion Sauce

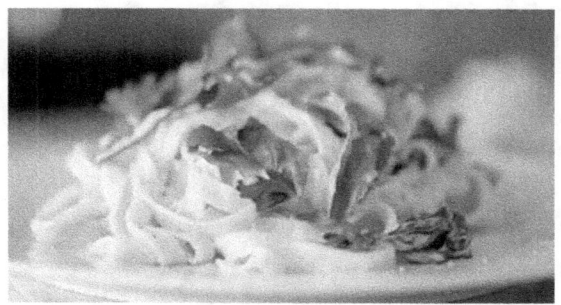

INGREDIENTS

Shallots – 2 pcs

Garlic bulbets – 2 pcs

Half of one avocado

Coconut oil – 5 gr

Olive oil – 20 gr

Basil leaves – 5-7 pcs

Juice of one lemon

INSTRUCTIONS

1. Chop shallots and mince garlic. Lightly fry in coconut oil

2. Put fried veggies, half of avocado, lemon juice, basil leaves, olive oil into blender. Blend for 2 minutes.

3. Use this creamy lemon, garlic and onion sauce with rice, grilled kale or brussels sprouts.

SALADS

7. Pork Salad (four servings)

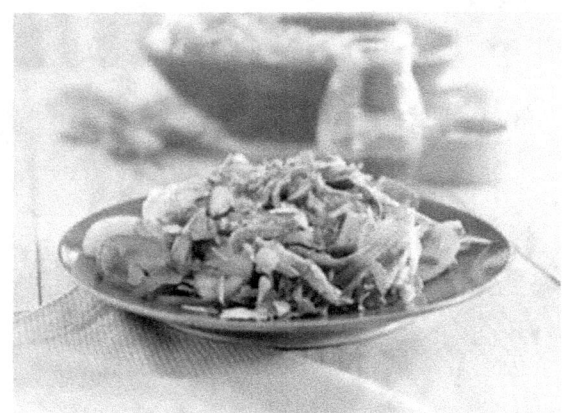

INGREDIENTS

Pork tenderloin – 450 gr

Olive oil – 36 gr

Cranberries - 1/2 cup

Shredded lettuce - 8 cups

Sliced cucumber – 1 cup

Slices of pineapple - 1 cup

Crushed walnut - 1/2 cup

Lemon wedges

Salt – 2,5 gr

Black pepper – 1 g

INSTRUCTIONS

1. Marinate pork tenderloin in salt and pepper.

2. Preheat oven to 180 C.

3. Lightly sear pork on both sides in olive oil. Then put it in a bakery dish and transfer to preheated oven. Bake for 15 minutes.

4. Take the pork out of the oven and let it cool down before you cut it.

5. Take a bowl. Put shredded lettuce on the bottom of the bowl and drizzle with olive oil and salt. Then put stripes of pork, slices of pineapple and cucumber, sprinkle with crushed walnuts and decorate the top of your salad with cranberries.

5. Better suited with lemon wedges. Enjoy!

8. Beet Salad

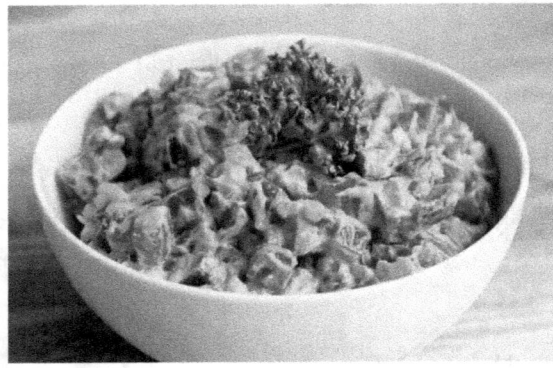

NOTE Beetroot is a very healthy vegetable. It is a great antioxidant! Beet is enriched with vitamin C and helps you to fight inflammation and reduce the risk of heart disease and cancer. In addition, beet improves digestion.

INGREDIENTS (four servings)

Coarsely grated beet – 450 gr

Coarsely grated carrot – 450 gr

Diced apple – 450 gr

Chopped almond – 60 gr

Garlic bulblets – 2 pcs (minced)

Perilla seed or pumpkin seed oil – 40 gr

Mixture of chopped parsley and dill

Salt – 1 gr

INSTRUCTIONS

1. Combine all salad ingredients together in a large deep bowl and mix.

Season with oil and salt.

2. Beet Salad is ready! Divide it into four servings and sprinkle with a mixture of chopped parsley and dill.

9. Kale Salad (four servings)

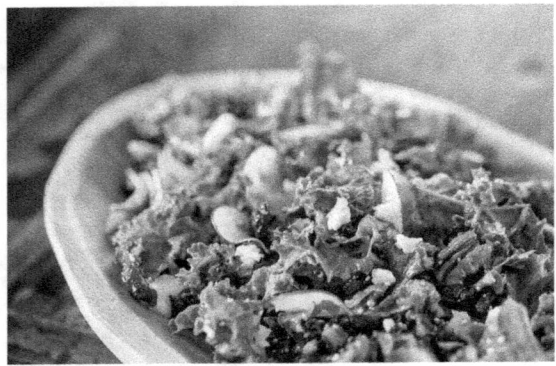

NOTE Kale is considered a low calorie product and known as "the queen of the greens", It is rich in fiber and it doesn`t content fats. In addition, kale is high in vitamin K, iron, antioxidants and omega-3 fatty acids. Add kale to you diet menu and it helps you to prevent inflammation and combat against such diseases as autoimmune disorders and arthritis and asthma.

INGREDIENTS

Kale – 6 cups

Extra-virgin oil – 18 gr (any you like – chia seeds oil, flaxseeds oil, olive oil, hemp seed oil etc.)

Chopped spring onion – 60 gr

Chopped red onion – 50 gr

Chopped Kalamata olives – 60 gr

Thin stripes of cucumber

Garlic bulbet – one piece (minced)

Half lemon

Dried basil

Pink rock salt or gray sea salt

INSTRUCTIONS

1. Wash the kale, dry it and cut into strips.
2. Steam kale stripes in a steamer basket for five-six minutes.
3. Take a deep bowl and put steamed kale into it. Season kale with dried basil, lemon, salt and oil. Mix carefully.
4. Add the rest salad components and stir again
5. Enjoy this delicious and healthy salad

10. Fruit Salad

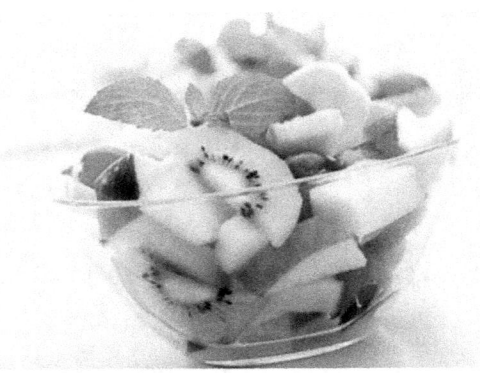

INGREDIENTS

Papaya – 1 piece

Half of one pineapple

Assorted berries - 3 cups

Apple – 1 piece

Juice and zest of one lemon

Juice of one orange

Almonds

Honey – 25 gr

INSTRUCTIONS

1. Wash, peel and chop papaya, apple, pineapple.

2. Take a small bowl and put there lemon zest, lemon and orange juice, add 25 gr of honey and mix thoroughly.

3. Take a large bowl and put chopped papaya, pineapple, assorted berries and chopped apple.

4. Pour liquid mixture in a large bowl and stir all ingredients together.

5. Decorate your fruit salad with sliced almonds.

11. Zucchini Salad

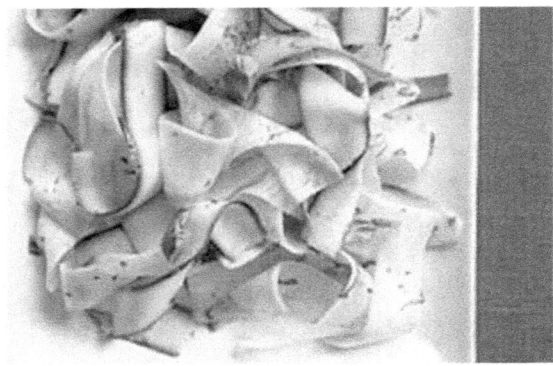

INGREDIENTS

Zucchini - 4 pcs (two yellow and two green)

Red chili pepper – 2 pcs

Lemon – 1 piece

Extra-virgin olive oil

Ground mustard – 5 gr

Sea salt

Sprigs of fresh basil – 1-2 pcs

INSTRUCTIONS

1. Wash zucchini, red chili peppers and lemon.

2. Peel zucchini into long thin ribbons, then finely cut the red chilies and put into a bowl.

3. Juice up the lemon. Take a mug and pour lemon juice and olive oil into it. Mix.

4. Combine ground mustard with salt. Season zucchini ribbons with liquid mixture and spices. Mix carefully.

5. Decorate zucchini salad with basil leaves.

6. Serve immediately!

AN ANTI-INFLAMMATORY LUNCH or DINNER

12. Pan Seared Salmon (two servings)

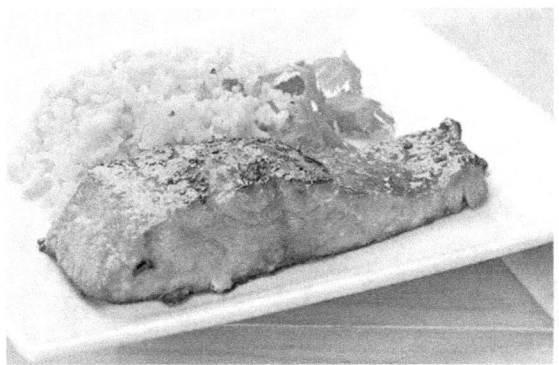

NOTE Salmon – is very healthy fish rich in Omega-3, bioactive peptides which may control inflammation in the digestive tracts. So, include salmon in your daily menu.

INGREDIENTS

Salmon fillets – 2 pcs

Lemon juice – 30 gr

Cherry tomatoes – 100 gr

Olive oil – 30 g

Salt, black pepper

Chopped baby arugula leaves – 3 cups

Chopped red onion – 40 gr

Extra-virgin olive oil – 18 gr

Red-wine vinegar – 18 gr

INSTRUCTIONS

1. Combine olive oil, lemon juice, salt, black pepper in a bowl. Marinate salmon fillets.

2. Heat the pan and put there marinated salmon fillets on it. Fry on both sides until crisp.

3. Slack the fire and cover the pan. Cook about three-four minutes.

4. Meanwhile, mix chopped arugula, red onion and halves of cherry tomatoes in a bowl. Season with oil and vinegar, salt and pepper to taste.

5. Transfer salmon on the dish and add vegetable mixture.

6. Bon appétit!

13. Grilled Salmon Teriyaki

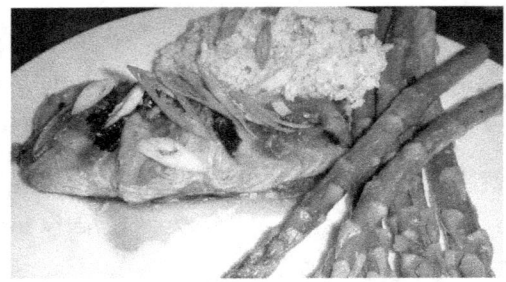

INGREDIENTS

Salmon fillets – 2 pcs

Teriyaki sauce – 45 gr

Ground black pepper – 5 gr

INSTRUCTIONS

1.Marinate salmon fillets in the teriyaki sauce for 10 minutes.

2.Put marinated salmon fillets on the grill and cook for 5-6 minutes on each side.

3. Serve immediately!

14. Turkey nectarine Burgers

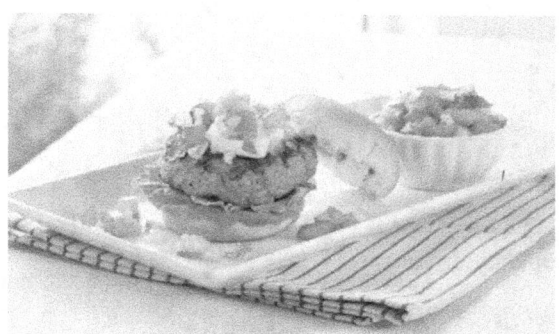

INGREDIENTS

Ground turkey meat – 450 gr

Onion – 1 piece

Nectarines – 2-3 pcs,

Dried tomatoes - 1/2 cup

Cilantro – one handful

Dried ground coriander – 25 gr

Sea salt (ground)

Pepper

INSTRUCTION

1. Prepare ingredients before start cooking. Finely dice onion, nectarines, dried tomatoes and chop cilantro

2.Lightly fry finely diced onion.

3. Take a deep bowl and place 450 gr of ground turkey meat and other components including fried onion.

4. Mix thoroughly.

5. Form medium-sized burgers. Refrigerate for 1-2 hours

6. Take burgers out of the fridge and grill on each side until cooked.

15. Herbed Chicken with Vegetables

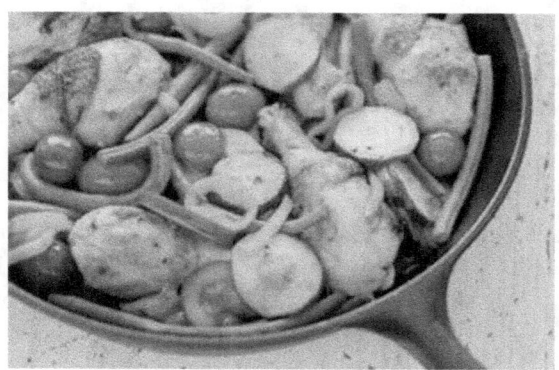

INGREDIENTS

Broiler – 1 piece (2 kg)

Chicken broth – 240 ml

Tomatoes – 2 pcs

Onion – 1 piece

Garlic bulbets – 2 pcs

Broccoli florets – 2 cups

Bay leaf – 1-2 pcs

Salt

Dried thyme – 10 gr

Pepper- 1 gr

INSTRUCTION

1. Wash dressed chicken, remove skin and cut up. Put it in a slow cooker.

2. Add chopped tomatoes, onion, and minced garlic into slow cooker.

3. Put 1-2 bay leaves, salt, dried thyme, pepper into the broth and pour over chicken.

4. Cook about seven-eight hours.

5. Add broccoli florets and cook one more hour.

6. Fragrant herbed chicken in its own juice is ready to eat!

16. Chicken Stir fry

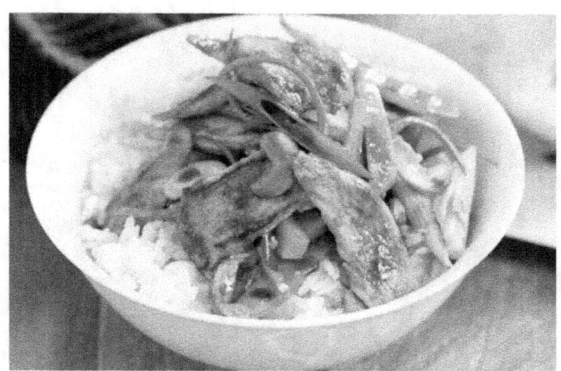

INGREDIENTS

Chicken breasts – 4 pcs

Half of one green pepper

Half of one red pepper

Half of one orange pepper

Half of one yellow pepper

Purple onion – 2 pcs

Red kidney beans – 1 can

Olive oil – 5 gr

STEP-BY-STEP INSTRUCTION

1. Wash, dry and slice all vegetables.

2. Wash and dry chicken breasts. Slice them.

3. Grease the pan with olive oil and fry slices of chicken breast until golden brown.

4. Add sliced vegetables, season with spices and herbs you'd like.

5. Let to stew in it`s own juice for 15-20 minutes.

6. Enjoy this fragrant dish!

17. Steamed Salmon with Lemon Scented Zucchini (four servings)

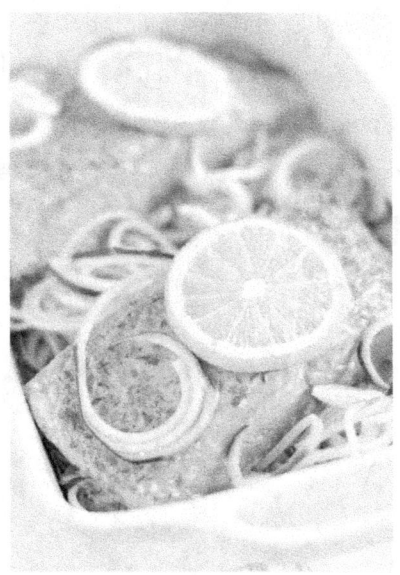

INGREDIENTS

Salmon fillets – 4 pcs

Sliced zucchini- 2 pcs

Sliced lemon – 1 piece

Sliced onion – 1 piece

Water 120 ml

White wine – 240 ml

Salt and pepper

STEP-BY-STEP INSTRUCTION

1. Put vegetables, water and white wine in the bottom of a Dutch oven.

2. Wash fish and dry with paper towel. Salt and pepper the fillets.

3. Grease the steamer rack and fit it over the vegetables in the Dutch oven.

4. Bring the liquid to the boiling point.

5. Slacken the fire and put salmon fillets on the rack. Cover and steam 10 minutes.

6. Serve fish on top of vegetable mix and liquid.

7. Decorate with olives.

18. Quinoa and Turkey Stuffed Peppers

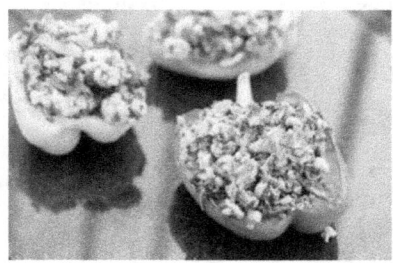

INGREDIENTS

Red bell peppers – 3 pcs

Uncooked quinoa – 1 cup

Diced smoked turkey sausage (fully-cooked) – 230 gr

Toasted and chopped pecans – 50 gr

Chicken broth – 120 ml

Water 480 ml

Chopped rosemary – 20 gr

Chopped parsley – 50 gr

Extra-virgin olive oil – 60 ml

INSTRUCTIONS

1. Take a saucepan. Put there uncooked quinoa, pour 480 ml of water, add salt and mix carefully. Bring this liquid mass to the boiling point.

2. Then slack the fire, cover the saucepan and stew until all water evaporates.

3. Meanwhile, combine diced smoked turkey sausage, chicken broth, olive oil, toasted and chopped pecans, chopped parsley and rosemary. Mix with ready quinoa mixture.

4. Preheat the oven to 180 C. Grease the baking dish with olive oil.

5. Take three red bell peppers, wash them and dry. Carve each pepper in two, remove peduncles, seeds and membranes. Cook pepper in boiling water for 3-4 minutes and then drain in a colander.

6. Stuff the peppers with the quinoa mixture. Place stuffed peppers on the baking dish.

7. Bake for 15 minutes at 175°C.

8. Take ready quinoa and turkey stuffed peppers out of the oven, put on a dish and drizzle with chopped greens.

9. Enjoy warm!

AN ANTI-INFLAMMATORY SOUPS

19. Pumpkin soup

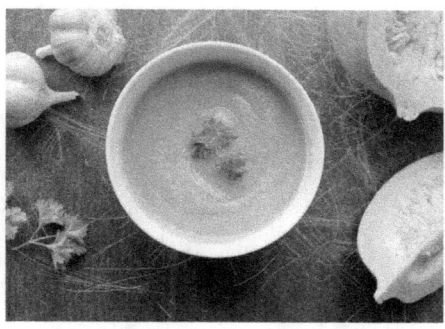

INGREDIENTS

Pumpkin puree – 1 l

Vegetable broth – 1,5 l

Onion – 1-2 pcs

Gingerroot – 11 cm

Almond milk – 120 ml

Garlic bulbets – 1 piece

Salt – 5 gr

Thyme – 3 gr

Fresh chopped parsley

INSTRUCTIONS

1. Peel and finely chop onion, garlic bulbets and gingerroot.

2. Add 240 ml of vegetable broth to spice mixture and simmer on low heat about 5 minutes.

3. Add remaining components (except parsley) and simmer for 30 minutes.

4. Whisk until smooth.

5. Drizzle with finely chopped parsley on top.

20. Cold Cucumber Soup

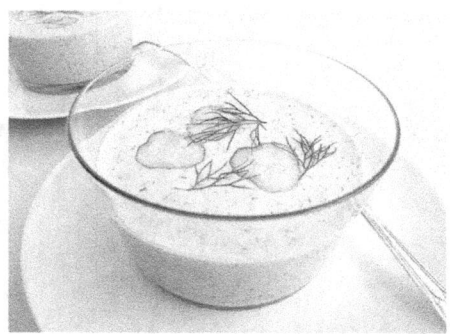

INGREDIENTS

Cucumbers – 6 pcs

Chicken broth – 360 ml peeled, halved lengthwise, seeds scraped out, and chopped

Fatless yogurt – 1 cup

Fresh parsley – 1 bunch

Fresh dill – one bunch

Juice of one lemon

Salt

Black pepper

INSTRUCTIONS

1. Prepare ingredients: peel, cut in length cucumbers, scrape out seeds and chop them. Take herbs (parsley and dill) and chop.

2. In a food processor or blender, Combine chopped cucumbers, parsley, dill, lemon juice in the kitchen unit and make puree.

3. Take half of the puree and half of the broth, add yogurt and mix.

4. Add this mixture to the puree in the kitchen unit. Blend again to mix completely.

5. Flavor with salt, pepper. Store in the refrigerator in a tightly closed container. 6. Serve cold!

AN ANTI-INFLAMMATORY BEVERAGES

21. Ginger Berry Smoothie

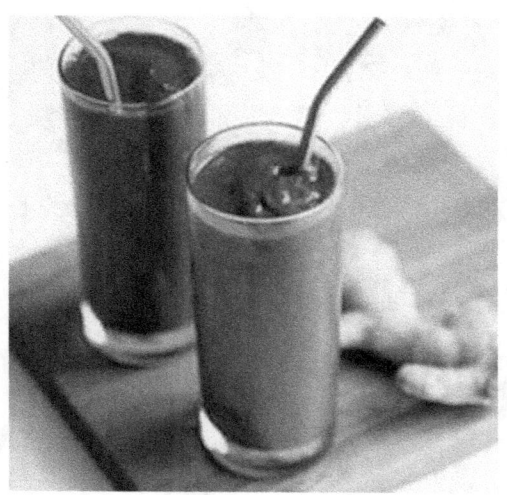

INGREDIENTS

Nutiva hemp protein powder – 90 gr

Peeled ginger – 5 cm

Celery – 1 cup

Leafy greens (any you like) – 2 cups

Assorted frozen berries (any you like) – 1 cup

Water – 120 ml

INSTRUCTIONS

1. Put all components in a blender. Blend until smooth.

2. Drink immediately!

22. Kiwi, Ginger and Banana Smoothie

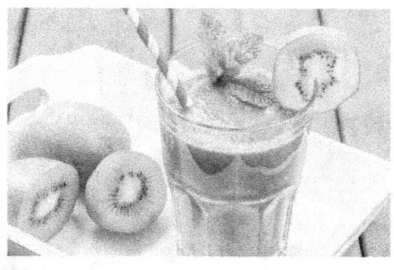

INGREDIENTS

Organic porridge oats – 36-48 gr

Kiwi – 3 pcs

Banana – 1 piece

Cube of ice – 8 pcs

Almond milk – 225 gr

Organic fat-free yoghurt – 240 gr

Ginger – 0,5 cm

Honey – 50 gr

INSTRUCTIONS

1. Peel kiwi and grate ginger.

2. Put all ingredients in blender (except honey).

3. Pour ready kiwi, ginger and banana smoothie in cups or glasses and season with honey

4. MMM! Yummy!

RECIPES OF ANTI-INFLAMMATORY JUICES

23. Purple Cabbage Juice

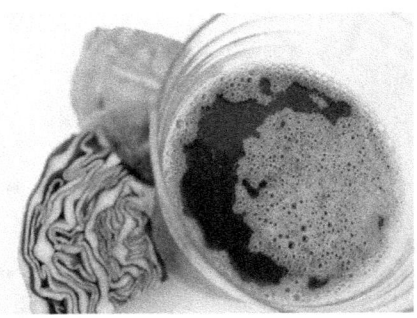

INGREDIENTS

Wedge of purple cabbage – 1 piece

Lime – 1 piece

Beet – 1 piece

Apple – 1 piece

Celery stalks – 6 pcs

Carrots – 6 pcs

Ginger

INSTRUCTIONS

1. Wash, peel and chop juice ingredients.

2. Juice them up, mix and serve!

24. Turmeric Vegetable juice

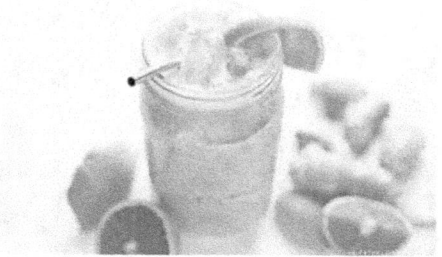

INGREDIENTS

Turmeric

Romaine lettuce -1 bunch

Carrots – 3 pcs

Cucumber – 1 piece

Lemon – 1 piece

INSTRUCTIONS

1. Wash, peel and chop juice ingredients.

2. Juice them up, mix.

3. Drink this turmeric juice when you're suffering from an infection!

25. Pineapple and Ginger Green Juice

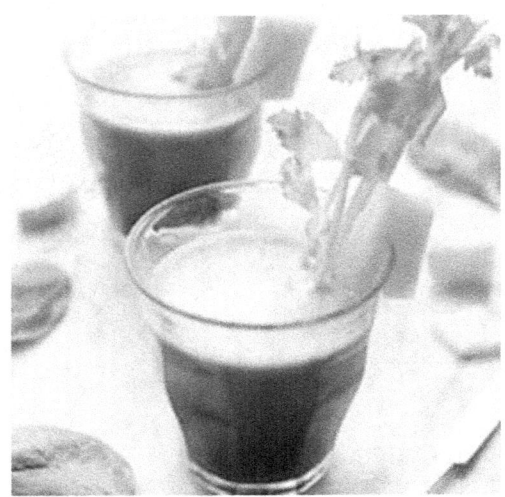

INGREDIENTS

Celery stalks – 4 pcs

Cucumber – 1 piece

Pineapple – 1 cup

Apple – 1 piece

Spinach – 1 cup

Lemon – 1 piece

Ginger

INSTRUCTIONS

1. Wash, peel and chop juice ingredients.

2. Juice them up, mix and serve!

26. Turmeric and Greens Juice

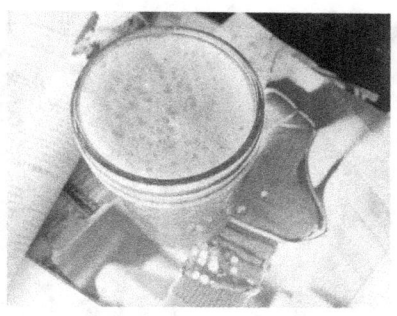

INGREDIENTS

Cucumber – 1 piece

Celery – 4 pcs

Lime – 1 piece

Oranges – 2 pcs

Spinach – 2 cups

Bunch of mint

Turmeric root – 2, 5 cm

INSTRUCTIONS

1. Wash, peel and chop juice ingredients.

2. Juice them up, mix and serve!

27. Spiced Carrots and Apple Juice

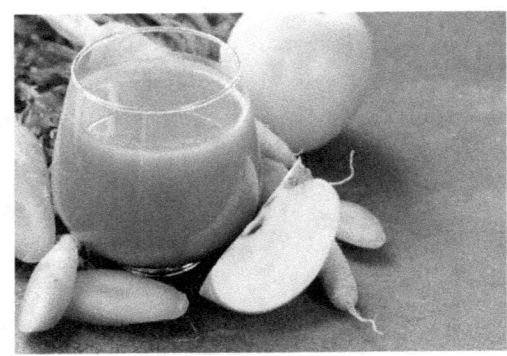

INGREDIENTS

Apples – 2 pcs

Carrots – 3 pcs

Celery stalks – 3 pcs

Ginger – 2,5 cm

Lemon – 2 pcs

Pear – 2 pcs

Turmeric root – 2 cm

INSTRUCTIONS

1. Wash, peel and chop juice ingredients.

2. Juice them up, mix and serve!

28. Citrus Juice with Flaxseeds

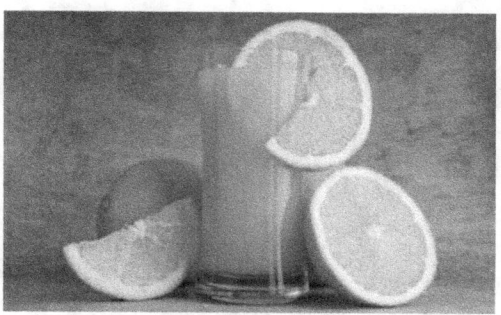

INGREDIENTS

Nectarine – 4 pcs

Lime – 1 piece

Lemon – 1 piece

Grapefruit – 1 piece

Ground flaxseeds – 25-30 gr

Turmeric – 10 g

INSTRUCTIONS

1. Wash, peel and chop juice ingredients.

2. Juice them up, mix and serve!

3. Add honey and ginger to taste.

29. Citrus Spice Juice

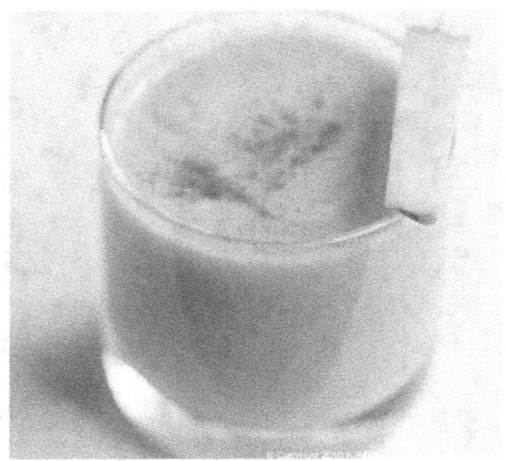

INGREDIENTS

A quarter of one pineapple

Yellow bell pepper – 1 piece

Celery stalks – 4 pcs

Yellow grapefruit – 1 piece

Ginger – 2 cm

Turmeric – 2 cm

INSTRUCTIONS

1. Wash, peel and chop juice ingredients.

2. Juice them up, mix and serve!

30. Seasonal Pumpkin Juice

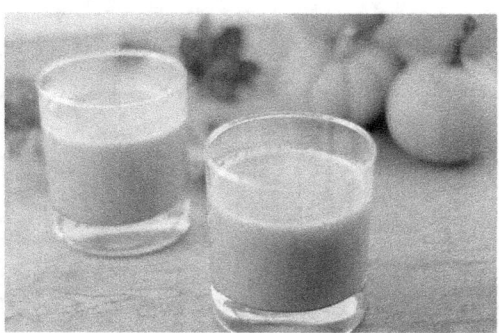

INGREDIENTS

Apple – 2 pcs

Half a butternut squash

Pumpkin pie spice – 10 gr

INSTRUCTIONS

1. Wash, peel and chop juice ingredients.

2. Juice them up, mix and serve!

31. Ginger Tea

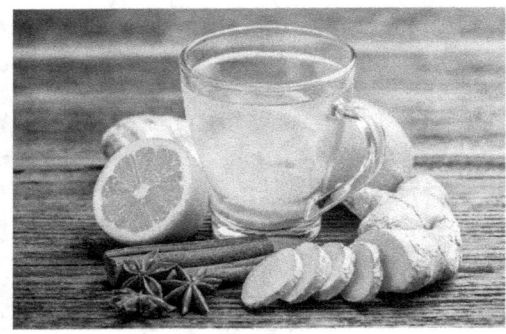

INGREDIENTS

Ginger – 5 cm

Water – 2, 5 l

INSTRUCTIONS

1. Take fresh ginger and peel it. Put in a kettle with water and boil for 25 - 30 minutes.

2. Let the tea to cool down.

3. Drink hot or cold as you like!

32. Lavender Lemonade

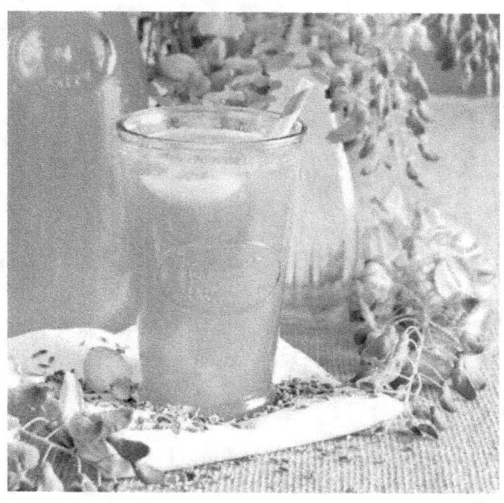

INGREDIENTS

Raw honey – 1 cup

Water- 1,2 l

Dried lavender – 35gr

Juice of 6 lemons,

Lavender sprigs

INSTRUCTIONS

1. Boil 600 ml of water. Add 1 cup of raw honey and 35 gr of dried lavender. Let brew for 25 minutes

2. Filter this flavored lemonade and pour into jug.

33. Turmeric Lemonade (four servings)

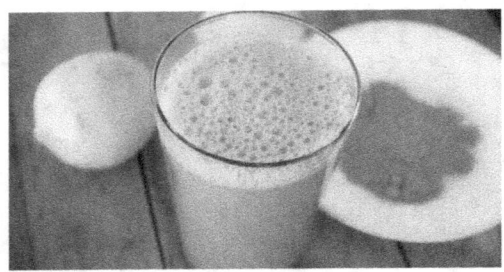

INGREDIENTS

Still or fizzy water – 1 l

Turmeric powder – 60 gr

Maple syrup – 70 gr

Juice of two lemons or limes

Juice of one blood orange

INSTRUCTIONS

1. Combine all ingredients together in a small jug,

2. Mix thoroughly and pour .into a glass.

3. Decorate glasses with lemon slices. Enjoy!

34. Dairy Free Oat Milk

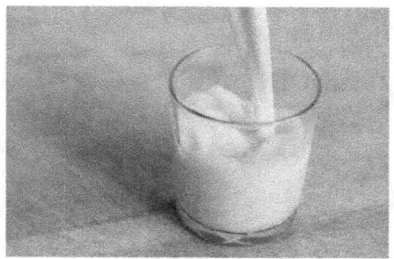

INGREDIENTS

Oats -1 cup

Cool water – 1,5 l

Sea salt – 1 gr

Cinnamon, vanilla, honey to taste

INSTRUCTIONS

1. Combine all ingredients together in a large saucepan, cover it and soak overnight.

2. In the morning blend this mass thoroughly for 2 minutes.

3. Filter the dairy free oat milk, add cinnamon, vanilla, honey to taste and pour into jug.

4. Store in the refrigerator in a tightly closed container.

AN ANTI-INFLAMMATORY DESSERTS

35. Oatmeal Banana Cookies

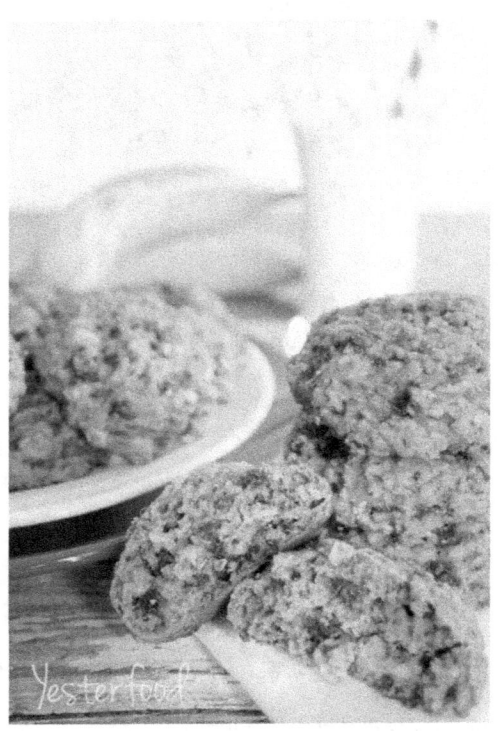

INGREDIENTS

Overripe bananas – 2 pcs

Quick oats – 1 cup

Applesauce – 3 gr

Crushed walnuts - 1/4 cup

Raisins - 1/4 cup

Cinnamon – 5 gr

Raw sugar – 6 gr

Salt

Coconut oil – 5-10 gr

INSTRUCTIONS

1. Turn on the oven and preheat it to 175 C.

2. Mash sweet overripe bananas. Add 1 cup of oats, 5 gr of cinnamon, 6 gr of raw sugar, 3 gr of applesauce, 1/4 cup of crushed walnuts, 1/4 cup of raisins and a pinch of salt. Mix thoroughly.

3. Grease the baking sheet with coconut oil. Form cookies with banana-oatmeal mixture and put on it. Your cookies may be flat or round (or any form you like).

4. You should have 16 cookies.

5. Bake oatmeal banana cookies for 35 minutes. Flip cookies and bake for another 10 minutes.

6. You're done! Remove cookies from oven and allow to cool.

7. Yummy! That tastes out of this world

36. Chocolate Walnut Treat

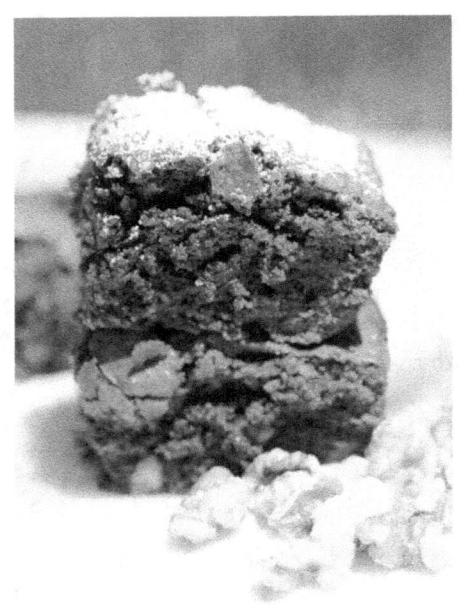

INGREDIENTS

Eggs – 5 pcs

Honey or agave nectar - 1/2 cup

Sea salt – 2 gr

Chopped black chocolate– 1 cup

Crushed walnuts – 2 cups

INSTRUCTIONS

1. Separate the whites from the yolks. Take a deep bowl, put egg yolks and honey in it. Whip.

2. In a separate bowl whip the egg whites and salt in a solid foam.

2. Combine the black chocolate-walnut mixture with the egg yolks mixture together. Then carefully enter the beaten egg whites into the mixture. Mix thoroughly!

3. Take a pan and grease it well with oil. Place mixture on the pan.

4. Bake at 175°C for 20 minutes, then switch off the oven and let this treat for 10 minutes.

5. Enjoy your chocolate walnut treat!

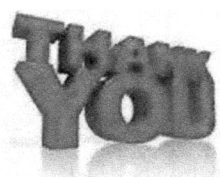

I am very happy that you have chosen this book and it's been a real pleasure writing it for you. My aim is to help as many readers as possible. So many of us are able to take new knowledge and use it to our lives with really useful and long lasting consequences and it is my desire that you have been able to take value from the information I have written.

Thank you for being with me during this book and for reading it through to the end. I really hope that you have enjoyed all the recipes and information I provided you and that's why I appreciate your thoughts on my material so much. If you could take a couple of minutes to write a feedback, your views will help me to create more material that you find beneficial.

Thanks again for your attention. I really look forward to reading your review.

Stay Healthy!

Sincerely, yours Rebecca.

Other Books Recommended by the Author

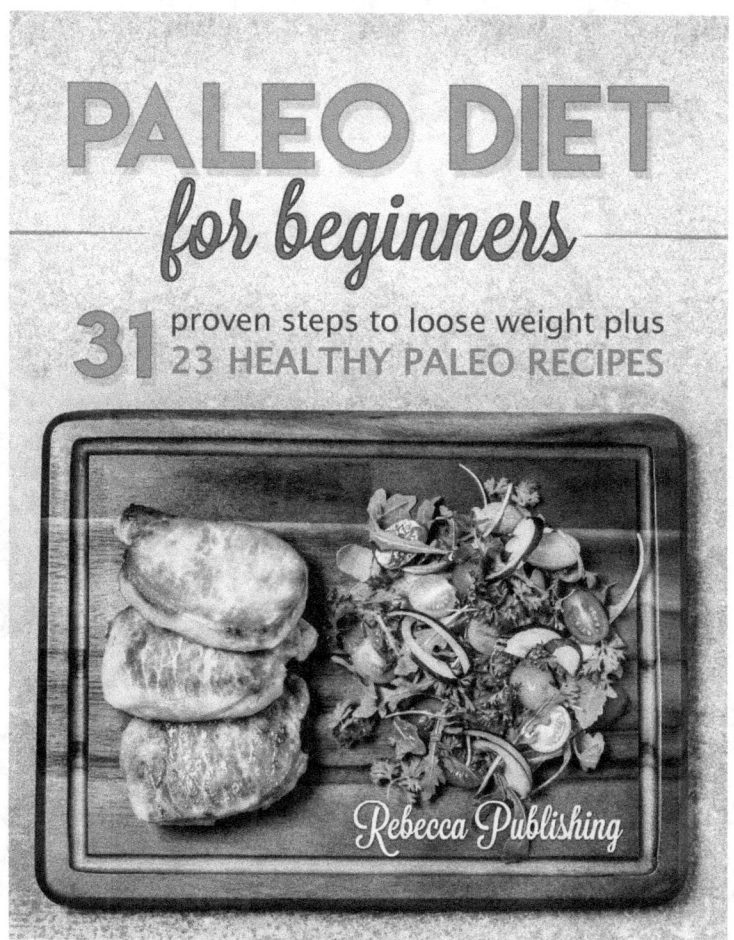

Please search this page over the www.amazon.com

www.amazon.com/s/ref=nb_sb_noss_2?url=search-alias%3Ddigital-text&field-keywords=B01MR9UU2O

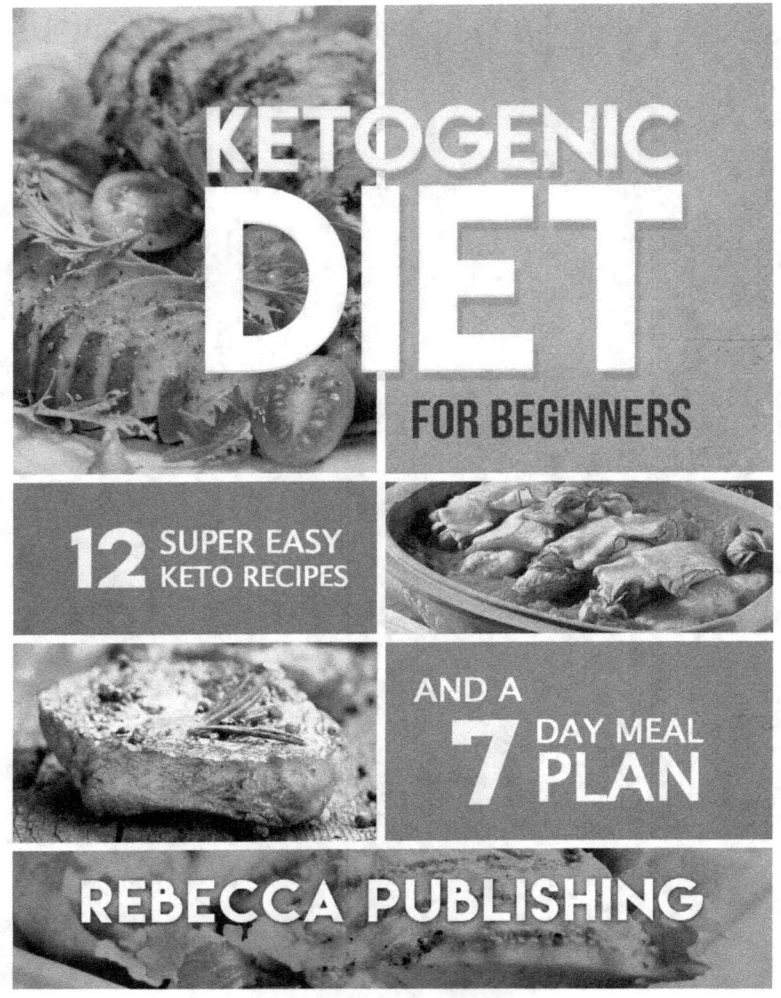

Please search this page over the www.amazon.com

www.amazon.com/s/ref=nb_sb_noss_2?url=search-alias%3Ddigital-text&field-keywords=B06XHQDK59

www.ingramcontent.com/pod-product-compliance
Lightning Source LLC
Chambersburg PA
CBHW081410280526
45788CB00009B/3047